An Ounce of Meditation

A tiny guide to get your started

Jenifer Cartland

Contents

Contents

Preface

The goal of this book is to introduce meditation in a clear, digestible way. There are many resources that go wider and deeper, but this book seeks to be a first, steady step through the door.

The title of this book reflects its size — it is an 'ounce-sized' introduction to meditation for those who are curious and who wish to explore this vast topic without getting tied up with a lot of complexities, commitments, or distractions.

The title is also meant to suggest something that research increasingly tells us is true — and that monks, yogis, meditators, and contemplatives of every stripe have told us for thousands of years — meditation is good for your body and mind. Medical research is beginning to conclude that 'an ounce of meditation' may be worth a pound of cure.

The meditation practices included throughout the book are by no means exhaustive. If any of these practices do not work for you, there are many, many others. These practices were chosen because they have worked for many people and are easy to share in a book like this.

I hope you enjoy this exploration and that, as your journey evolves, you find a meditative practice that brings you peace of mind and body.

Acknowledgements

Even 'tiny guides' like this one take inspiration and support from others in order to move them from a vague idea to a book with words, chapters and a cover. I am deeply grateful to my many yoga teachers over the years who in small ways and large opened my eyes to the power of meditation, and helped me find simple words to describe my experiences.

Of my teachers, I want to recognize the excellent faculty at Yoga North International SomaYoga Institute, especially Ann Maxwell and Molly McManus, whose kindness and open-heartedness continues to help me find my path. I am also indebted to Angela Farmer, who truly walks the talk of yoga practice and models the power of a consistent meditation practice in her word and deed.

Several colleagues and friends read versions of this manuscript and offered helpful insights, found problems, and fixed mistakes that made the book better. These are Danielle Foertsch Newman, Kami Nixon, Chris Schlapper, and my husband, Jeff Sader. I am so profoundly grateful for their friendship and, in the case of Jeff, for his seemingly boundless love and support.

Finally, many of my students and clients have taught me how best to offer meditation to them (and how NOT to offer it). Their willingness to share their experiences and continue the conversation with me shapes every page of this small book. I look forward to our continued learning together.

What is meditation?

During meditation, you focus your attention and eliminate the stream of jumbled thoughts that may be crowding your mind and causing stress. (Mayo Clinic)

[Meditation] is the cessation of the fluctuations of the mind. (Patanjali, The Yoga Sutras)

At its most simple, meditation is a way to give your mind a rest while remaining awake.

Our bodies get excited when our minds are excited. When your mind rests, your body is more able to rest.

Sometimes it is helpful to meditate about something. But meditation is not problem-solving or active thinking. It is an attempt to hold your mind in a restful state while remaining awake.

It can be difficult, but simply trying to meditate is often enough to begin to feel its effects. Most of us never really get past the 'trying' stage. So don't fret about becoming an expert at meditation. It is something to try over and over. And as you try, it will start helping you.

Your mind, all the time

Many of us leave our windows open all the time,
allowing the sights and sounds of the world to invade us.
(Thich Nhat Hahn)

Your mind's job is to keep you safe. It does this by problem-solving in big and small ways. It does this by worrying. It does this by organizing to-do lists. It does this by bringing information in from the world around you tirelessly. The mind is very, very busy. That is its job.

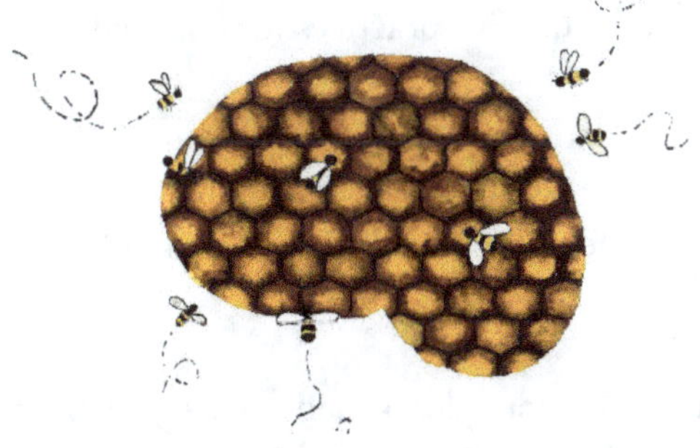

The mind can be like

- a three-year-old who cannot sit still
- a teenager the night before she takes her SATs
- a parent with a dozen to-do lists
- a library filled with books that need to be constantly sorted and shelved

It works all the time. And that is a good thing. Did you know your brain uses 20% of all your calories? That is a lot for such a little lump of flesh!

The mind is never bad or wrong for working so hard. In fact, we should thank it for keeping us safe!

But sometimes the mind gets too active. And when that happens, your heart can race, your breath can become rapid and shallow, and you can feel miserable. You can feel like you are out of control.

By practicing meditation, you learn how to close the windows. You learn how to calm the mind, to give it a time out, and to gently restart its engine, your engine.

What doctors say

Meditation is an ancient practice. Thousands of years ago, yoga practitioners experimented with ways of calming the mind. Many religions have used meditative practices for hundreds and thousands of years.

Over the last thirty years, medical researchers have started studying meditation and its effects. So far, they have found that by meditating:

(1)   Your anxiety is reduced
(2)   You can think more clearly and solve problems better
(3)   You can adapt to changes more fluidly
(4)   You can sort through emotions more effectively

Also:

(5)   Your blood pressure goes down
(6)   You sleep better
(7)   Your heart works more effortlessly

(8)   Your brain works efficiently

(9)   Your brain ages more slowly

Lots of good things!

Is meditation religious?

Meditation need not be religious. It works for everyone, regardless of their beliefs. However, most religions have 'contemplative' practices that use meditation techniques. For many people, prayer can be meditative.

But if prayer is worried or panicked or about figuring something out, it is not a form of meditation. Prayer may lead to meditation, but it is not meditative until your mind pauses its work. That is the key. The brain needs to take a break. Resting in contemplative prayer can be a lovely way to do that. Thomas Merton, a Roman Catholic monk, called contemplation 'a dialogue of deep wills.'

Meditation practice #1: Tell your brain to stop

Many people try to begin practicing meditation by 'controlling' the mind or telling it to stop working. Let's try that.

Find a comfortable sitting position. Take a couple settling breaths. Ask your mind to pause. Give it three minutes.

Watch the activity of your brain. Notice, if you can, what comes up for you, how long thoughts stay, how many there are and how well you can rest your brain.

How did that work for you? Did you feel like your mind rested?

Most meditators believe that this approach to quieting the mind is either impossible or only for the most advanced meditators. The mind's job is to work. All the time. So telling it to stop is pretty impossible. Your mind simply does not understand 'Stop.'

Meditation practice #2: Give your brain a stick to hold

There is a famous account of elephants being marched through markets in India. They caused chaos by sampling every piece of food they could lay their trunks on. But their handlers learned that if they gave the elephant a stick to hold with their trunk, the elephant would focus on the work of holding the stick and lose interest in other things. They could then walk calmly through the marketplace.

That is what we are going to try first. We are going to give your brain a stick to hold.

Focus your attention on one of these things (your brain's stick):

- Your breath going in and out (breathe through your nose)
- A candle flame (in your mind or a real flame)
- Imagine waves coming and going on the shore

Just watch the breath or the flame or the waves as long as you can.

You will likely find that your mind wants to go back to working. That is ok. After all, that is its job. Just bring your mind back to your breath or the candle or the waves. Be patient, be kind. You are teaching a sweet, little, energetic, confused three-year-old to sit still. He does not understand why you are doing this. He does not know it is good for him.

Here are a couple more helpful tips to keep your mind focused:

Thich Nhat Hahn, a Buddhist monk who wrote and taught a lot about meditation, suggested saying this to yourself -

I am breathing in. The breath goes in.
I am breathing out. The breath goes out.

Repeat this over and over as you meditate. And when you stop saying it because your mind wanders, come back to saying it again.

Pema Chodron, a Buddhist nun who also has written and taught a lot about meditation, suggests another technique. She suggests identifying thoughts as what they are (that is, your mind being active) and then letting them go. When a new thought comes into your mind, say, 'Thinking!' and let the thought go. Return to your breath or the candle or the waves.

It is important to not get aggravated at how active your mind is. Be kind. Be thankful. It is just doing its job. But also be persistent. Three-year-olds need to learn to sit still, at least a little.

A soft landing

Many people have a hard time sitting with their minds, especially as they begin their meditation journey. This box offers a practice that anyone can be successful with. If you struggle with any of the practices in the book, feel free to come back to this one. It is meant to restore you, to relieve frustration, and to help you unshackle any difficulties you are having with meditation.

As we will see in the coming chapters, rather than being calming, meditation can act as an echo chamber for whatever is worrying or frustrating us. That means that meditation can be difficult, even uncomfortable and scary. Research shows that people who are anxious or depressed, for example, have a harder time with solitude than others because they have negative thoughts that get louder and repetitive in solitude. Thus, activities that pull them out of solitude may feel more comforting (listening to music or the tv, being with friends, doing 'busy' work, etc.).

In the 1970s, Rachel and Stephen Kaplan (both psychologists) posited that nature can be mentally soothing for individuals under certain circumstances. They wanted to find ways to help people refresh the energy of what they called 'spent attention' -- the feeling of exhaustion you feel after doing particularly demanding mental work.

Research since then has explored the concepts of soft and hard 'fascination' in this context. Hard fascination is directed thinking of some kind (learning, planning, paying your bills), the kind of thinking that might wear you out. Soft fascination is a kind of non-directed thinking in which your mind is infused with awe. It is refreshing. It fills your tank.

Many of us experience soft fascination when we are in nature, which is what the Kaplans observed. But we can also feel it at art museums, in cathedrals, and in many other places. It comes upon us when our minds are gently active, when we are observing the world around us in a relaxed way and the feeling of awe comes over us.

Another characteristic of the experience of soft fascination is connectedness. Often, when a person experiences awe, they experience an expansive connection to all the things around them, such as nature, animals, or other people.

Since most of us have had soft fascination experiences, we can remind ourselves of these soft fascination experiences at any time. We can relive them. Indeed, many guided meditations encourage meditators to return to soft fascination experiences they have had in the past by asking them to imagine themselves in a forest, or to imagine the sound of gentle rain fall. It is a great place to start and to return to.

A soft fascination exercise

Bring to mind experiences you have had of awe when you were in nature or in the presence of something that spurred a feeling of awe. Choose one experience that has especially vivid or heart-felt memories.

Close your eyes and try to remember as much as you can about that experience. Bring to mind smells, sounds, and sights. Allow yourself to be emersed in the memory.

Hold that memory for as long as you like. Perhaps notice how this memory feels in your body and mind. Notice how you feel when you have held the memory for a few minutes.

Soft fascination experiences are not exactly meditation, but they are a very close cousin. Enjoy these. Use them to refresh yourself and your mind. Always feel free to return to this exercise when other meditation practices are not sitting well for you. They are a soft landing, always waiting for you.

Your breath and meditation

One conscious breath, in and out, is a meditation.
(Eckhart Tolle)

The breath is a bridge between the body and mind.
(Swami Rama)

Your breath is a unique and wonderful thing. It speeds up when you need it to and slows down when you are relaxed. It supplies just the right amount of air so your body can keep working. And it does this without you having to worry about it. But that is just part of what makes your breath so special.

Our brain sends signals to all of our body parts to keep them working, to speed up, to slow down, and to sleep. We are not even aware of most of these signals. Even so, the brain churns on and on, and keeps the whole system going.

But unlike other organs of the body (like the liver and the stomach), the lungs can also be controlled by conscious effort. We can tell our breath to slow down or speed up.

So our breath is controlled by *two* processes, not just one — most of the time, our brain sends signals to our breath without us being aware *and*, sometimes, *when we want to,* we can consciously tell our breath to speed up or slow down. And when we decide to calm our breath, the rest of our bodies and our minds listen and become calm, too.

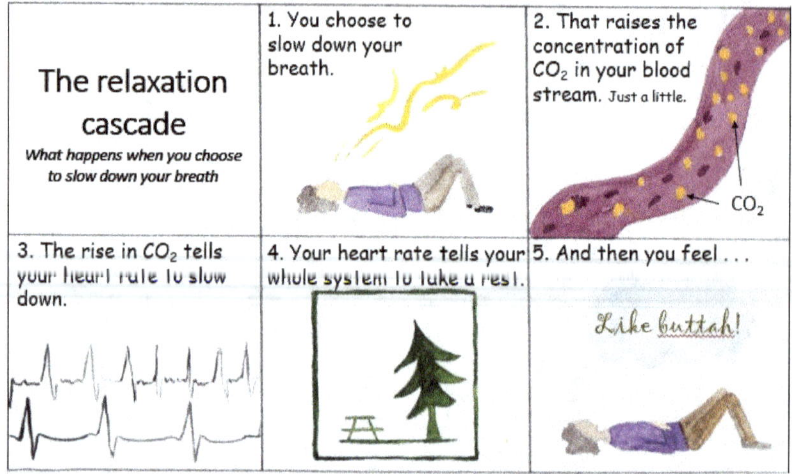

This is what makes the breath unique, and also what makes it especially wonderful. We can use the conscious control of the breath to bring our whole body into a more restful state. It can 'down-regulate' our entire nervous system.

Try it! The next time you are nervous, anxious, or just out of sorts, pause and breathe out slowly. Breathe in through your nose. Purse your lips and pretend you are breathing out through a straw. Do it a few times. You will notice that your whole system settles down. Your heart rate slows, your breath becomes deeper and softer, and your mind calms.

Meditators often use breathing exercises to calm the mind. Your breath is an amazing and effective tool at the ready to give your mind a helping hand.

Meditation practice #3: Triangle and square breath

Many people find that trying to control the breath makes them uncomfortable and nervous. If that is what you feel when you go through this exercise, no problem. Just skip it. You can come back to it later, or just use other tools. There is no law that says you need to have a breath practice to meditate. But many people find it helpful.

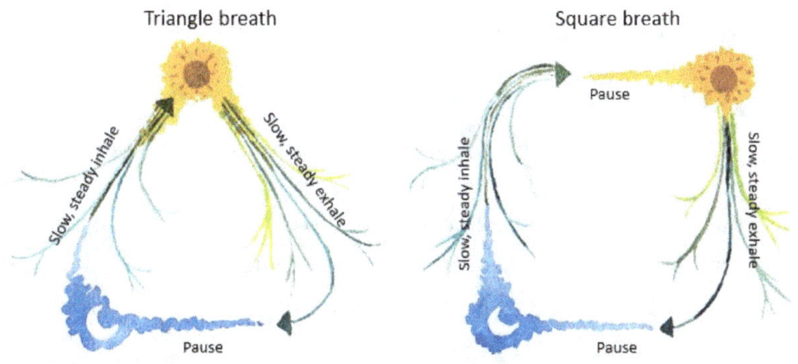

Sit upright or lie down on your back. If you are sitting, sit in a chair or on some blankets on the floor. Your spine should be in a neutral position. You want the airway to be clear and at ease. Breath through your nose.

Notice your breath. As you do this, your breath will become more regular.

Scan your body and mind. How do you feel? Anxious? Relaxed? Uncomfortable? Exhausted? Happy? Simply take note of those feelings.

Take a number of these breaths and allow yourself become calm.

Notice your breath. As you do this, your breath will become softer, longer, and deeper.

Now notice that at the top of your breath (when your lungs are full) there is a tiny pause before you let the breath out. And at the bottom of the breath (when your lungs feel empty), there is another tiny pause.

Thus, the breath has four parts, not just two - we breathe in, we pause, we breathe out, we pause.

Let those pauses happen. Don't try to control them, don't worry about them. Just notice them.

You can continue breathing with this awareness for as long as you like.

Triangle or 3-part breath: Another option is to explore elongating the pause after your out-breath. Don't try to hold the breath. Don't allow yourself to feel air hunger. See if the pause can get longer. Maybe it can, maybe it can't. Just explore.

Square or 4-part breath: Finally, you may choose to explore elongating the pause that comes naturally at the top of the in-breath as well as at the bottom of the out-breath. No holding your breath; just pause and explore the stillness.

Scan your body and mind again. How do you feel now? Do you feel any different as a result of this breathing this way? Simply notice.

How to breathe deeply:

Start by breathing normally and explore if your breath is moving into your abdomen. When you breathe, your diaphragm presses down into your abdomen, pushing all of your organs out of the way. Is this happening?

There is often a lot of tension in the belly. That is where our 'fight or flight' response begins. And for many of us, that response can be 'on' all the time, as if we are always ready for the next shoe to drop.

If there is tension in your belly, the diaphragm cannot move easily and your breath will not be deep, it may even feel rushed or jagged. So try to see if you can gently nudge tense spots into being softer.

As your belly softens, your breath will naturally deepen. Imagine how a dog, cat or baby breathes – they use their whole trunk. Try to be soft enough in your belly (all the way down to your pubic bone and hip joints), your sides and your lower back so that your diaphragm has great ease when it moves.

If you can't get rid of tension in your belly, that's ok. Just let the movement of the breath rock the edges of the tense areas. They will soften in time.

Your emotions and meditation

Meditation . . . [develops] devotion, compassion, and the ability to forgive. (The Dalai Lama)

When people begin to meditate, emotions often surface that surprise them. This may happen to you. Here are a few ways emotions can surface through meditation:

- You may resist meditating. You may have a vague feeling or discomfort that you cannot pin down.
- During meditation, a memory may pop up. It may be very intense. You may be filled with joy, sadness or some other emotion you can't even name. You may not understand it right away.
- As you begin to meditate more, you may be surprised to find that you get less riled up by certain things that used to get under your skin.

Yes. These things happen sometimes. Indeed, here is what Thomas Merton said of his own contemplation experience:

Contemplation is no pain-killer. What a holocaust takes place in this steady burning to ashes of old worn-out words, cliches, slogans, rationalizations!

What is happening here? Isn't meditation supposed to make everything better?

At the beginning of this book, one of the definitions of meditation given is from Patanjali. He is considered the 'father' of yoga. This is what he said:

[Meditation] is the cessation of the fluctuations of the mind.

In other words, meditation is a way to quiet the mind and all the things that disturb it. Emotions are one of the things that can disturb the mind. They can really get the mind riled up.

Patanjali calls emotions 'seeds' that are planted in our minds over time. Many, many emotions and memories lie deep in our minds as hidden seeds of thought and action. Thomas Merton uses the exact same imagery.

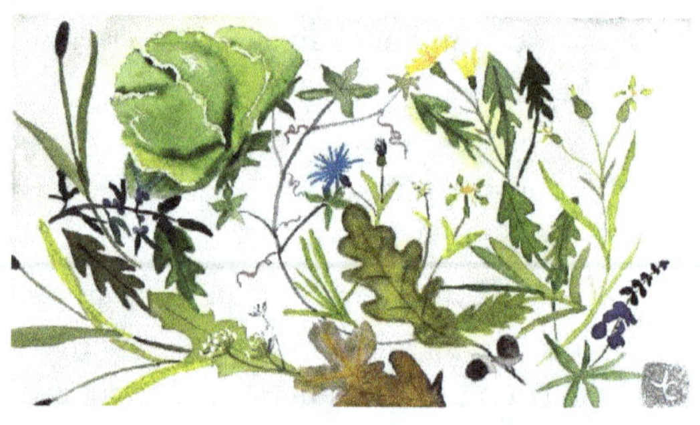

Meditation clears your mind of all the other things that you normally think of during the day, and that can give these seeds space to get a little sunlight again, maybe even to sprout and grow.

What are these seeds? They can be anything. Have you ever flown off the handle at a small thing and not really understood why? There was probably some emotional memory that got triggered. Maybe it was a memory of the way your dad scolded you once or the way the weather was one day or car trouble you had years ago. It could be anything. But there you were shouting at someone who did not deserve it.

This happens to everyone. It is often these hidden, forgotten seeds that sprout when we least expect them. They often seem to come from nowhere. They often feel uncontrollable.

And one place they show up more clearly than in other places is in meditation.

According to Patanjali and Merton, this is ok, and should be expected. Meditation is a safe space where you cannot hurt anyone else's feelings.

But you can hurt your own feelings, so let's look a little more deeply.

Meditation helps us become aware of emotions, even powerful ones, for the first time in a long time. Sometimes, we may even 'see' these emotions for the first time ever. This can be frightening. In meditation, it is possible for childhood memories, small hurts, giant wounds that we thought were all tucked away, to wave their hands at us as if to say, 'I need some help here!' They can be positive and warm us with a deep inner smile that seems to come out of the blue, or they can be very hard to face – as Thomas Merton called them, a 'holocaust' of emotion.

Meditation gives us the space to explore these emotions simply as thoughts that affect our minds and bodies (and hearts). Once we see them this way, we can converse with them like other thoughts and sensations and make decisions about what to do with them. Maybe we do nothing with them. Maybe we let them sit for another day. Maybe we learn more about them. It is up to us.

Emotions can be intense. So go slow. You may not be ready to deal with something the first time it pops up. Lower your expectations. Be kind to yourself. Be patient, persistent, and positive.

The good side of this

As these seeds sprout and we converse with them, many, many old hurts and wounds have the opportunity to *heal*.

This is what Patanjali wanted to see, and what the Dalai Lama was saying in the quote that headed this section. It is incredibly good for us. It helps us behave more mindfully with those we love and with the wider world. We spread less hurt to others because we have fewer unintentional outbursts. We become kinder, more empathetic, more patient. We are less afraid.

Thomas Merton says that when we work through these things, all that is left is the 'existential altar of what *is*.' Erich Schiffman, a highly-regarded yoga teacher, puts it this way:

> *Love is what is left when you let go of everything you don't need.*

It is scary, but it is good, helpful work.

Meditation practice #4: Notice emotions

Sit quietly and allow your mind to come into quiet. Begin to watch your breath and allow your mind to calm down with your breath. Breathe through your nose.

Now, bring up a good memory -- something that makes you feel safe and comfortable. Explore the sensations in your body and mind. How does this memory make you feel? What is happening to your breath? To your heart rate? To your heart?

Now, bring up a memory that is less pleasant -- something small, like forgetting something on the grocery list or a minor disagreement with a loved one. Notice shifts in the sensations in your body and mind. Take a few breaths here. Just notice. What is happening to your breath, to your heart rate? To your heart?

Come back to your safe and pleasant memory. Breathe. Let that linger a bit until you feel calmer and at peace again.

Emotions play rough and tumble with our minds, bodies and hearts. Meditation can help us see how these unpredictable seeds sprout and grow, and gives us some space to sort things through in our own time.

Your brain and meditation

The mind is definitely something that can be transformed, and meditation is a means to transform it. (The Dalai Lama)

The regular practice of meditation can change the physical structure of the brain and create positive changes in mood and behavior. (Eileen Luder, PhD, Neuroscientist)

In the last several years, research has started to move quickly towards what we all hope will be important breakthroughs for people who suffer from or are at risk for neurodegenerative disorders (like dementia and Parkinson's disease). And meditation looks as though it may play a starring role.

There are additional breakthroughs for individuals that struggle with anxiety, depression and attention deficit and hyperactivity disorder (ADHD), and that support the use of meditation in managing those conditions.

I am going to break down the current thinking so that you can explore the best way for meditation to work for you.

Brain waves and meditation: The basics

Electrical currents/oscillations (what are commonly called 'waves') in the brain are responsible for all nervous system activity. There are five types of waves. All five types of waves are active all the time, but depending on what activities you are engaged in, one will be dominant. The brain switches between these wave forms instantaneously and seamlessly based on what you are trying to do.

The five types of waves differ in three ways: (1) Their speed, (2) their size (amplitude), and (3) the part of the brain in which they are most active.

The table below details the types of waves and how they relate to meditation, based on the scientific consensus over the last 20-30 years.

Wave type	Speed	Part of brain where it is most active	What the brain is doing when this wave form is dominant
Gamma	35-40 Hz	All parts of the brain	Taking new information in, connecting the dots, integrating new information with old
Beta	12-38 Hz	Parietal and frontal regions	Awake, alert, engaged; motor control
Alpha	8-12 Hz	Occipital region	Quiet, contemplative, passive attention; meditation
Theta	3-8 Hz	Parietal and temporal regions	Day dreaming, dreaming in sleep; deep meditation
Delta	.5-4 Hz	Cortex	Deep sleep; deep meditation

As you can see from the table, the meditating brain is dominated by slower wave movement in general. Today, research is a bit unclear about which waves are most dominant during meditation. It appears related to the depth of the meditative state, the experience of the meditator and their ability to maintain that state for some time.

In the ancient yoga texts, there is a notion that one must maintain certain states for 10 or 20 minutes to BEGIN to enter the deepest meditative states. Meditators may agree with that, but research so far is undecided. What we do know for sure is that the experience meditators have of slowing down their systems is validated by research. Research is just unclear about how MUCH meditators can slow down their brain activity.

The rest of this chapter explores the implications of slowing down the activity of the brain.

Anxiety, depression and ADHD

The brain has five 'lobes,' or five large regions. Within and between those regions are many, many smaller areas and connections. Recently, neuroscientists have developed the idea of 'large neural networks' by studying the combination of wave activity in different regions of the brain while individuals are engaged in different sorts of activities.

A large neural network is a group of parts of the brain that become active together, and that get quiet together. A network could involve parts of two or three different lobes of the brain and the connectivity between them. For example, when you are working intensely on a task, the 'executive control' network is activated. The executive control network involves eighteen sub-regions of the brain. These regions coordinate your tasks so that you can smoothly move from one activity to the next. Other parts of your brain are relatively quiet during these times.

In the 1990s, researchers noticed that when individuals were relaxed and not 'on task,' certain parts of the brain were very active and other parts quieted down. This network is called the 'default mode network' (DMN). It is the network of brain activity that operates when we are not doing anything purposeful. These non-purposeful activities may include mind-wandering, ruminations, day dreaming, undercurrents of worry -- any brain activity that does not require focus.

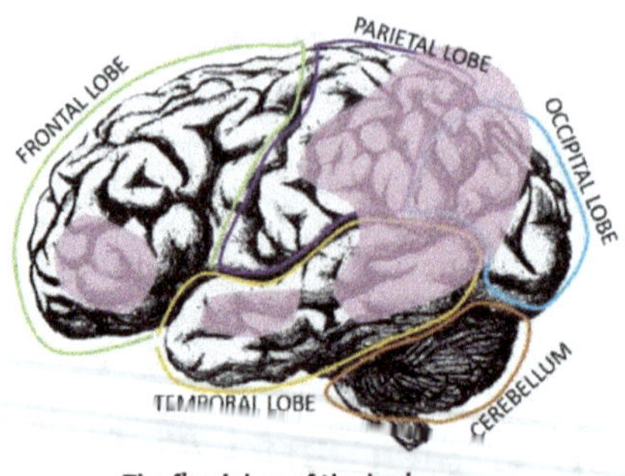

The five lobes of the brain
and the default mode network
(DMN, in pink)

In the last several years, research has looked at the DMN in the context of anxiety, depression and ADHD, all conditions where non-purposeful brain activity appear to play a heightened role. The general conclusion of this research is that when an individual experiences these mental health concerns, their DMN is 'over active.' It is like the idle on their brain motor is set higher than when they are not experiencing these symptoms.

Earlier, it was noted that individuals with these conditions can find solitude especially hard because quiet can amplify their negative thoughts. The higher idle on the DMN may be responsible.

Research is now showing that meditation reduces DMN activity both during active meditation and AFTER the meditation session has concluded, making it a great management tool for some of the most common mental health concerns. It brings down the idle on the brain's motor.

How might this work? Let's presume you have anxiety disorder (it is the most common mental health concern, with about 20% of US adults experiencing it each year). As a result, your brain ruminates often about worries that perhaps other people would take more lightly. And the worry just won't leave you alone. It may even lead to panic attacks or sleeplessness.

By meditating, you may be able to slow down the pace of the DMN and thereby reduce the frequency and power of your ruminations — quiet down the echo chamber. Meditation would become, then, one of the several tools you use to manage your anxiety. Very promising!

Neurodegeneration

The second big area of research around meditation and brain health focuses on neurodegeneration, problems that occur as we age. Many parts of our body function differently as we get older, and the brain is no different. The most prevalent neurodegenerative disorder is Alzheimer's disease.

A number of factors are at play in the development of neurodegenerative conditions, such as genetics and behavior choices over many years. The research community has studied the build-up of certain types of waste material in the brain in the elderly, which has been hypothesized to be a trigger for some forms of neurodegeneration (notably Alzheimer's and Parkinson's diseases). The way waste material builds up may be related to genetics and behaviors, but the bottom line is that, for all older people, it builds up to some degree.

The issue is not the presence of waste material per se because waste material just happens as part of living. The issue is that as we age (or as a result of significant injury), our ability to clear the waste from the brain is reduced. The result is that waste builds up day after day and that build-up can cause lots of problems. Many researchers view the reduction of cleansing activity as a key pathway for the development of neurodegenerative disorders.

Brain health during aging: New research

Since 2012, there has been an explosion of information about how the brain takes care of itself, and the potential role of meditation. Prior to this time, research consistently showed that long time meditators suffer fewer neurodegenerative disorders than others. The new research sets the stage for a fresh look at the precise relationship between meditation and brain health. Here are the key findings:

(1) The brain has a special system to clear waste materials from its tissue, called the glymph system. The glymph system was discovered in 2012. It works in deep sleep when brain activity is dominated by the slowest brain waves (delta waves).

(2) Delta waves during deep sleep have been shown to actually squeeze/pump out the waste.

(3) As you age, you get less of this deep sleep every night. Young adults spend about 20% of their sleep time in deep sleep. Older adults spend 2-8% of their sleeping time in deep sleep. It is not altogether clear why older adults get less deep sleep, but we know they do.

Therefore, the current theory is that because aging individuals get less deep sleep than younger folks and because deep sleep is critical to waste clearing in the brain, older individuals become more susceptible to neurodegenerative diseases that stem from poor waste release from the brain. It seems like a snowball effect may be triggered, with less deep sleep reducing waste clearing, and lack of waste clearing being one of the potential reasons for poorer sleep. We have a lot more to learn.

The trend towards less waste clearing would happen to all aging individuals. But for some individuals, because of injury, genetics, behaviors or many other things we do not yet understand, the clearing slows down too much. As a result, neurodegenerative symptoms begin to surface.

This is the current theory supported by a growing body of research (see the section *Further Reading on the Science of Meditation* for more resources). We all have waste products that build up in our brain during the day. Deep sleep clears them. Older people get less deep sleep, so they are vulnerable to the disorders that the build-up of waste can cause.

Meditation and brain health

Additional research is needed in order for the medical community to start recommending meditation for mental health concerns (although many clinicians do recommend it, especially for anxiety), and before meditation is recommended as prevention for neurodegenerative disorders (although, as with anxiety and depression, some clinicians do already).

The one thing we know for sure is that our understanding of the role of meditation in managing the activity of the brain is expanding, and so far it explains why long-time meditators experience fewer problems as they age. Through meditation, meditators activate slower brain waves, which would help clear waste from the brain.

This does not mean meditation is the cure-all, but certainly it would seem to be an activity that could help us manage several mental health conditions that make life hard for us (anxiety, depression and ADHD) and could help us stack the odds in our favor when it comes to neurodegenerative disorders.

Meditation practice #5: Reducing the negative chatter

Preparing for this practice

If you find your mind to be quite talkative when you try to enter meditation, it is useful to prepare for meditation by moving a bit. A traditional yoga practice may be a lovely way to quiet the mind by giving the body work to do, and meditation sessions are typically held at the end of yoga classes for that reason. An alternative is to simply take a walk.

The goal is to discharge some physical energy so that you are not dealing with pent up 'wiggliness'. My mother used to tell her five children to run around the house three times when we got home from school. Once I became a mother and watched my kids explode with energy after sitting in school all day, I understood this for the first time. They simply could not sit down to do homework without releasing the physical energy that built up in their muscles and bones all day. So give yourself that release.

Sometimes, after a physical energy release, the mind will find a quieter, less chattery place on its own. If you find that to be true for you, you can then choose to try any of the practices offered in this book.

If your mind is still chattery, especially if the chatter is negative, overrun with ruminations, or anxious thoughts, an additional set of tools may help.

A practice for an anxious and fearful mind

First, I want to acknowledge that the anxious and fearful mind is quite a challenge to quiet down. So prepare for the hard work and choose a 'soft landing' in case meditation does not seem to work for you. Have the soft landing in your pocket as back up. It will leave you feeling positive and refreshed no matter how your meditation practice goes.

In this practice, we are going to set a 'sankulpa' (san-KUHL-pah, a connection to the highest truth). A sankulpa is a positive intention that we will 'seed' into your meditation practice. It is similar to a mantra, but the goal of the sankulpa is joy and healing.

There are two rules for an effective sankulpa.

1. A sankulpa is always expressed in the positive. For example, if you want to set an intention about eating better, your sankulpa could be 'It is easy to eat well' or 'I show love for myself with food choices.'
2. A sankulpa is always expressed as if it is already true. For example, 'I *am* kind to myself,' not 'I *will be* kind to myself.'

Step 1: Begin by thinking about the message you need to hear when you are frightened or anxious. Jot a number of these down. Don't try to make them perfect. Just jot down what comes to you. Take your time here.

Step 2: Once you have some ideas of words that comfort you, try to rephrase each set of words in positive and present terms. Instead of 'everything always works out,' you might write 'everything IS working out.' Instead of 'everything will be ok,' write 'everything IS ok.' Instead of 'hurts will heal,' you might write 'I am healed.'

It is not important that you believe that your positive and present sankulpas are true right now. Indeed, you may not believe them at all. The goal of this practice is *to shift them into true* in your heart and in your mind.

Step 3: So now you have a couple of sankulpas to try out. Pick one to try first. Try this sankulpa in meditation a few times. You will know if it is working for you, or if it needs to change. Once you find a sankulpa that sits well with you, stick with it for several months, even a year. Sankulpas are seeds we sow for the long haul.

Sowing your sankulpa

Note that this practice has a number of steps, and you might find it confusing. The bottom line is to anchor your practice around these five steps:

(1) Settling into the practice through the breath.
(2) Repeating your sankulpa three times.
(3) Scanning your body and letting go.
(4) Repeating your sankulpa again.
(5) Coming out of the meditation gently.

Take your time with each of these stages. The practice should take about 10 minutes. What follows is one more detailed version that may be helpful.

The full practice:

Find a comfortable position to meditate. This might be one that feels best lying down. Whatever position you choose, find comfort. You will be in this position for 8-10 minutes.

Perform the following steps in sequence, with deliberation. Take your time.

(1) Come to your breath. Notice your breath moving in your body.

(2) Focus on your outbreaths. Make them longer. Count down from 10 to 1 with each outbreath. As you count down, you will feel your body soften further.

(3) Bring to mind your sankulpa. Repeat it three times in your mind.

Be positive. The work is already done. You are your true self. You are luminous, whole, uninjured.

(4) Turn your attention to your body. Scan your body. Imagine points of light at each joint. Move your mind from one joint to the next. Let go.

(5) Feel your body to be heavy. Let gravity pull on you. Notice the weight of your body on the floor or in your chair.

Notice the weight of your head, your shoulders, your pelvis, your legs, your heels.

(6) Feel lightness. Feel that space between your body and the floor expand, maybe just a millimeter or two. Feel that expansion.

Feel yourself light, floating. Stay floating as long as you like.

(7) Rest for a moment now. Just breathe.

(8) Repeat your sankulpa three times. The work is already done. You are your true self. You are luminous, whole, uninjured.

(9) Rest. When you are ready to be finished, invite more breath into your body and gently begin to move again.

Your experiences of pain and meditation

Meditation is not evasion, it is a serene encounter with reality. (Thich Nhat Hahn)

Bring your attention to the pain as if you were gently comforting a child, holding it in a loving and soothing attention. (Jack Kornfield)

We have all heard stories of yogis who could walk on beds of hot coals without feeling pain, or yogis who have kept themselves alive and hardy in weather that would cause hypothermia in humans who do not have decades of yogic training. We are not talking about this kind of heroics here. We are going to stick close to the science for ordinary people, acknowledging that pain is an important source of information to our bodies, and we are going to explore how meditation can help us cope with it.

Over the last twenty years, meditation has been shown to be a useful tool in the management of pain. And more recent research is beginning to understand how this is so.

Pain is one way your body tells you something is wrong and that it needs attending. Once you understand the cause of pain and are attending to it appropriately, meditation can be part of the pain relief strategy.

Pain comes in two forms: Acute and chronic. In the case of acute pain (you just broke your wrist, you have kidney stones, or your appendix is infected), your first job is to fix the injured or unhealthy body part. That will relieve pain eventually. During the process of getting relief for acute pain, meditation may offer some relief to bridge you through. But getting attention to the injury or illness is the most important thing to do.

Chronic pain lasts more than three months or after an injury has healed completely. Unlike acute pain signals, chronic pain signals are not very precise. In fact, they can be quite complicated. In the book *Pain is Really Strange*, neurologist Steve Haines explains that (a) our brains may get 'trained to pain,' and give us pain signals long after a pain source has healed, (b) pain signals can be 'referred' to or from a different part of the body, or (c) pain signals can recur at the mere suggestion of the stimulus that caused the first injury, in the case of some trauma responses. In all of these cases, the body's tissue is as healthy as it can be, but we receive incorrect signals that it is not healthy.

The pain cycle

A lot of the aches and pains folks complain about are chronic but not constant and fit into the 'healed but still feels vulnerable' category. For example, many years ago, a disc in my low back was injured. Currently, my low back feels just fine, but after a few hours in the garden, low back pain sometimes kicks up. So it is most correct to say I have chronic low back problems and recurring pain, but not constant pain. It has been decades since my disc issue occurred and all of the tissues involved are now healed as much as they ever will be, but nonetheless, recurring pain is a reality for me.

The chronic pain cycle points to the need for movement in the treatment of chronic or recurring pain. Lack of movement weakens muscles and bones and destabilizes joints, which will make pain worse, and perhaps allow it to spread to other areas in the body. Therapeutic movement will restore functionality while reducing the recurrence of pain episodes. The body is meant to move. And movement is part of the healing process.

For me, yoga practice has been a significant source of healing and of building the resilience in areas of my body where recurrent pain occasionally shows up, like my low back. But it does not need to be yoga. Movement is always better than non-movement, if you can move at all.

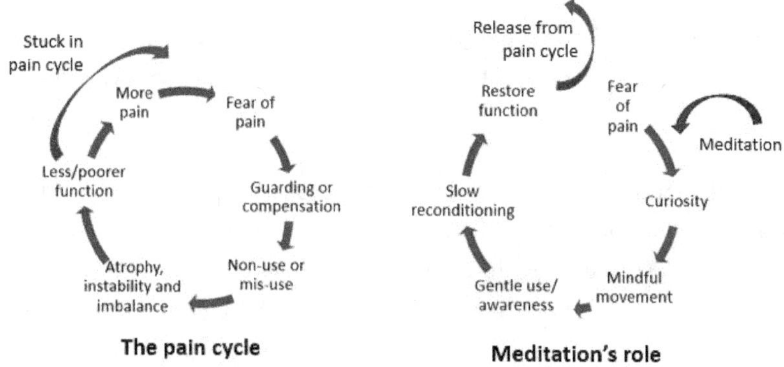

Where does meditation fit in?

As I have already stated, meditation practitioners can use meditation as a partial bridge for acute pain until medical care has been delivered and the illness or injury has healed. Natural childbirth advocates who focus on breathing techniques have long pointed this out. And meditation can help with chronic pain, even for folks who are new to meditation.

When your body experiences pain, 'nociceptors' (neurons that specialize in observing pain) send a signal to your brain that there is a problem. Meditators, research shows, feel these signals, but they experience them less severely and are less likely to rate these signals as 'very unpleasant.' What that means is that meditation keeps us in touch with the needs of our bodies, but we react less dramatically.

This is worth emphasizing. Meditators do not 'disassociate' and ignore pain signals. Disassociation is a response that the mind makes under extreme trauma. It is a survival mechanism. In disassociation, the individual's mind stops feeling physical pain because the pain is unbearable. There are unfortunately human experiences where this is a needed survival mechanism.

But meditation does not rely on this mechanism. Meditators do not disassociate. Meditators feel the physical pain, but less intensely. And they see it as <u>less</u> unpleasant than others (it is still unpleasant, but perhaps not overwhelmingly so).

That little bit of mental space perhaps opens the capacity to be curious about the pain rather than afraid of it. The meditator might ask HOW the painful area feels (tingling, buzzing, or pulling, for example) and WHEN the pain changes or becomes worse (while moving gently, under emotional stress, or shifting one's body to a new position).

Once curious, meditation may give us the capacity to keep moving when others may feel incapacitated, fearful or overwhelmed by the pain. If you keep moving, you heal faster and build resilience against future injury.

Research shows that meditators experience about 30% less pain than non-meditators, which for some conditions and some individuals (everyone experiences pain differently) is enough to reduce the use of pain medications and/or to stay consistent with therapeutic movement. Managing pain while using fewer pain-reducing medications is a win. Getting back on your feet quickly after a recurring injury knocks you out for the seventeenth time is also a win.

As an example, one of my yoga teachers is in her mid-80s and has been practicing yoga for over sixty years (which for her has always included meditation practice). She has experienced her share of physical bumps and bruises throughout her life and as she has gotten older. In a recent class, she challenged us to think of pain as 'just' another sensation that can be helpful and informative, and not something to push away.

It occurred to me as she spoke that she has reached a sort of acceptance with the ordinary physical aches and pains of aging. She uses this acceptance to help her work with her painful places more effectively, to heal more quickly and to stay more resilient. Her curiosity opens the capacity to work WITH the pain, not AGAINST it.

The good news is that you do not need a sixty-year meditation practice to achieve this pain relief. Research shows that even new meditators can learn to work with their pain with curiosity rather than fear.

The added benefit of long-term meditation

New meditators and long-time meditators both benefit from the 30% reduction. But long-time meditators have a different cognitive reaction to pain, and maybe this is what my yoga teacher was trying to encourage. For new meditators, there is essentially a dampening of the pain signal coming to the brain. Long-term meditators' brains react to pain differently.

The brains of long-time meditators (>1000 hours of practice) observe the same intensity of pain, but find the pain to be significantly less disturbing. MRI studies show that the portions of their brains associated with *sensory discrimination are more active* and the portions of their brains focused on *emotional appraisal are less active* compared to non-meditators and new meditators (<10 hrs of practice). This shift from emotional reaction to sensory exploration enables a mental shift in which the experience of pain is decoupled from the emotional reaction to the pain. Long time meditators have the capacity to shift from fear to curiosity.

Recall that my yoga teacher counselled us on exactly this point – to show curiosity and ask what the pain can teach us, to let the pain guide us, rather than become overwhelmed and fearful. My teacher might agree with Ram Dass, who said, "Once you start to spiritually awaken, you re-perceive your own suffering and start to work with it as a vehicle for awakening."

Buddhists use the concept of 'the second arrow.' The first arrow wounds you. The second arrow is your reaction to the wound, and it can cause more damage than the first wound itself. Thus, we can see, both metaphorically and physiologically, how long-term meditation helps us avoid or manage the 'second arrow' of an injury or illness. It remaps our brain's responses to pain and decouples the experience of pain from the emotional response to it. This allows us to evaluate the pain and our reaction to it with curiosity and creativity rather than fear or feelings or helplessness. Modern research appears to have verified what Buddhists and yogis have told us for centuries.

30% is not 100%

Finally, I want to emphasize that a reduction in pain is not the elimination of pain. Pain continues to be an important part of how our bodies speak to us, and we need to stay open to it. We also need to be honest with ourselves when pain needs medical attention and when meditation and other home practices can offer sufficient support. Every individual experiences pain differently, and we need to let our own bodies lead the way. There is no shame in getting help from a medical provider. It is simply that meditation can help, too. It is another tool in your belt.

Meditation practice #6: Managing the information flow

This practice is designed to heighten your awareness of sensory information and explore your ability to let go of it. It is intended to build the mental muscle to help you cope with discomfort.

Find a comfortable position to meditate. This might be one that feels best lying down. Whatever position you choose, find comfort. You will be in this position for 8-10 minutes.

Take each step one at a time. There is no rush to finish this. Even doing just half of this can be valuable.

(1) Close your eyes and come to your breath. Notice your breath moving in your body.

(2) Focus on your outbreaths. Make them longer. Count down from 10 to 1 with each outbreath. As you count down, you will feel your body soften further.

(3) Bring your attention to your skin. Notice how some of your skin is warm, some is cold, some may feel pressed against the chair or floor. Just notice and pause here for as long as you like. Let that noticing go. Come back to your breath.

(4) Bring your attention to your mouth. Notice the feel of your tongue, soften your upper palate. Notice any tastes, any sharpness, and temperature differences. Just notice and pause

here for as long as you like. Let that noticing go. Come back to your breath.

(5)   Bring your attention to your nose. Feel the air coming and going. How does the air feel? Cool, warm, damp? Are there smells you can find? Don't try to figure the smells out. Just notice them and pause here for as long as you like. Let that noticing go. Come back to your breath.

(6)   Bring your attention to your ears and to any sounds you may hear in the room or outside the room. Scan your space for sounds, not to figure them out, but to simply bring them to awareness. Just notice them and pause here for as long as you like. Let that noticing go. Come back to your breath.

(7)   Bring your attention to the part of your mind that gives attention. For most people, that is a spot between and a little above their eyebrows and an inch or so deep. Notice the vibrations of that spot. Notice how it sits still or does not. Just notice and pause here for as long as you like.

(8)   Rest.

(9)   Bring your attention back to the part of your mind that gives attention. Let it wake up.

(10) Bring your attention to your ears and the sounds around you.

(11) Bring you attention to your nose and the movement of your breath in your nostrils.

(12) Bring your attention to your mouth and any tastes or sensations it offers you.

(13) Bring your attention to your skin and all of the sensations it provides for you.

(14) Bring your attention to your breath moving in your belly. Bring in more breath. Allow your body to gently waken.

Your immune system and meditation

Nature does not hurry, yet everything is accomplished.
(Lao Tzu)

Here is something new and exciting: physicians now believe that meditation helps our immune system. As if meditation did not already have plenty of other benefits, now there is one more, and a big one to boot!

The movement of lymph fluid

This part is a little technical, but may help you visualize the connection between the immune system and breathing.

Diaphragmatic breathing is when you use your respiratory diaphragm to breathe – when all of the organs in your belly move. There is a long, narrow duct that runs vertically inside the ribcage. It is called the thoracic duct. Material is pumped up through that duct when you breathe diaphragmatically.

That material is called 'lymph' – fluid that carries 'stuff' our cells do not need out of our bodies (for example, lymph fluid carries viruses, bacteria, and things that cannot be absorbed into the blood stream).

Lymph fluid comes from everywhere in the body. It pauses at the lymph nodes, gets cleaned up a bit, and then travels to our kidneys where it leaves our system.

	Blood circulatory system	Immune 'circulatory' system
Fluid that circulates	Blood	Lymph fluid
Force that moves the fluid	Heart beat	Muscle movement, diaphragm
Pace of fluid movement	5-6 liters per MINUTE	3-4 liters per DAY
Direction of fluid movement	Fluid moves into and out of the body tissues	Moves fluid OUT of the body tissues only
Main organs	Heart, lungs, bone marrow	Lymph nodes, spleen, thymus

Lymph fluid coming from the upper body travels through ports near your collar bones, and drains into a vein connected to your kidneys. Lymph fluid that comes from below the ribcage (your abdomen and legs) gets pumped up through the thoracic duct in your ribcage by your respiratory diaphragm, and then joins the lymph fluid from your upper body in the vein that carries it to the kidneys.

Compared the circulatory system, in which blood is pumped by the heart through the body, the immune system uses muscle movement to collect and transmit the lymph fluid into the waste system. As mentioned, the respiratory diaphragm does a key part of the pumping — it moves fluid from the lower half of the body up the thoracic duct so that it travel to the kidneys. Hence, the importance of diaphragmatic breathing for the immune system.

Two ways meditation may help

Meditation, researchers think, does two things that help the immune system. First, it deepens our breath.

Meditation often includes breath practices, and so it helps you breathe better – it helps you develop and use diaphragmatic breathing techniques. The better you breathe, the better the lymph fluid moves. And the better the lymph fluid moves, the better you can fight infections.

The second way meditation helps the immune system was covered in the section *Your Brain and Meditation*. The glymph system in your brain is activated by slowing down the brain waves. The cleaning action works best when the brain is at rest or you are asleep. And what do you do when you meditate? *You rest your brain.*

As mentioned in the previous chapter, studies have found that long-time meditators suffer fewer neurodegenerative diseases. These are diseases, such as dementia, where the brain loses function as we age. Much of the loss of function is from injurious substances that don't get cleaned out of the brain as much as we wish they did.

The current thinking is that meditation helps the brain's immune system clean out unnecessary 'stuff' and keep the brain functioning optimally.

An ounce of meditation is truly worth many pounds of cure, it seems.

Meditation practice #7: Move that lymph!

Any kind of movement helps lymph move through your system. We are going to focus here on using the breath in a specific way that helps the lymph move up the duct in your ribcage. And by quieting our minds while we do it, our brains can have a little cleaning time, too.

Move into a comfortable seated position or lie down on your back. Find your breath. Soften the space between your ribs and your hip joints. Scan that space for areas of tension and explore whether the movement from the breath can bring softness to those areas.

We are going to take three long, soft, slow breaths. On the first inhale, try to keep all the areas above your belly button still and allow your breath to move all the areas below your belly button, including your lower back and sides.

On the second breath, hold your chest still and allow the breath to move everything below the ribs, including your back and sides — all the way down to your hip joints — but have the feeling of starting at the pubic or hip joints and filling from the bottom up.

On the third breath, starting at the pubic bone, allow movement all the way up to your collar bones.

Repeat this sequence of three breaths five times, while using your calm, steady breath to quiet your mind.

Meditation practice #8: Walking meditation

Like diaphragmatic breathing, any movement of your main joints moves lymph toward your kidneys. (Note: The lymph-like fluid in the brain operates best when we are at rest. That is the opposite of the lymph movement in the rest of the body, which moves best when our bodies move.)

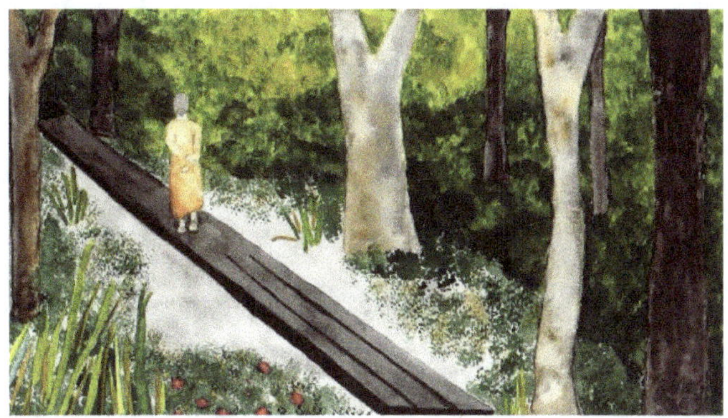

Find a space indoors or outdoors. You need a space at least about 15 feet to walk. You will walk quite slowly back and forth in this space, so consider a surface that will allow you to be balanced and comfortable.

If you feel out of balance, dragging your fingers along a wall or a kitchen counter, or using a cane or a walker can help steady you.

Here is how you do it:

(1)   Situate yourself at the end of your walking space, facing the other end.

(2)   Slowly begin to lift your right foot. As you do, say 'lifting, lifting, lifting.'

(3)   As you move your foot forward, say 'moving, moving, moving.'

(4)   As you move your foot to the ground, say 'dropping, dropping, dropping.'

Repeat with your left foot. And then continue across the space, repeating the 'lifting, lifting, lifting,' etc. with each foot movement.

When you reach the end of the space, you need to turn around.
Follow this process:

Bring your feet together, turn your right foot 90 degrees, bring your
left foot to meet it. Turn your right foot another 90 degrees, bring
your left foot to meet it.

You are now turned around and ready to walk the length of your space
again.

Make every movement with kindness and deliberation.

Your meditation practice

I have so much to do today, that I must meditate for two hours instead of one. (Gandhi)

Discovering compassionate self-discipline may be easier and harder than you thought. (Cheri Huber)

Keep up your meditation, as there is no instant illumination. The mind moves slowly in this. (The Dalai Lama)

Now that we have explored some basic facts about what meditation is, how to do it, and how it helps you, it is time to think about whether you would want to put a practice together for yourself.

Are you wondering where to start? Here are some questions to consider:

(1) How long will you meditate? Try different lengths of time and see how it works for you. After a week, do you feel more stable during the day with 10 minutes a day? If so, you are on the right track.

(2) Will you use a timer? It gives your brain one less thing to wrestle over while you are meditating. Set the timer on your

phone or in your kitchen. The *Resources* section reviews a few apps that can be helpful in developing a practice. There are many, many apps. The ones offered here are simply ones that I have used.

(3)   Will you meditate every day? Most meditators like the daily habit. They find it grounds their day and sets them up to manage whatever slings and arrows come their way.

(4)   Will you keep track of your meditation sessions? If you are the kind of person who likes checking things off a to-do list, it might help to put a reminder on your phone and check the box when you finish each day. Or keep track on a sheet of paper. Some templates are offered here in the *Resources* section. If checking boxes and keeping track makes you crazy, don't do it.

(5)   Will you keep a meditation journal? Many people find a journal a helpful way to track what might come up for them in meditation. Some journalling templates are offered in the *Resources* section. But if it becomes a chore and prevents you from sitting in meditation, choose meditation over journalling.

(6)   Will you combine meditation with other activities? This is a question to ask yourself. Many runners and yoga practitioners feel that they enter a meditative state during these activities. That is great. But also keep in mind that a lot of runners think about becoming better runners when they run, and a lot of yogis think about holding poses better when they do yoga. In meditation practice, your mind's rest is the priority. If you cannot make it a priority when you are doing these other things, then keep meditation separate and enjoy these other activities for the wonders that they are.

My basic advice is to start with a 5-10 minute morning practice for three weeks, which is the time it generally takes to establish a habit. On the day before you begin, choose a time, a length and a place. Then start, and repeat it every day for three weeks. Don't try to perfect your time, place or length right now; that can be a distraction. Simply settle into a routine.

If meditation works for you, after the three weeks, your body/mind may simply wake up each day and say 'do meditation!' or you will crave it when you miss a day, or you will say, 'I would rather do this in the other room or outside or after I shower.' And then make the change and stick with that.

Finally, there is no person or god in heaven, on earth or anywhere else who is judging your meditation practice. It is yours. It is for you. If it brings you joy, do more. If it makes your life better, do yourself the favor of being consistent with it. If you stop meditating because life gets in the way, start again. That is the practice – just starting again.

Be patient, persistent and positive. All will come with practice.

Resources to support your practice

Inspirational teachers

These are teachers I have grown to love. There are many, many books and guides out there, and many are excellent. But I have personally found all three of these very helpful.

Pema Chodron, *How to Meditate: A Practical Guide to Making Friends with Your Mind.* Chodron is a Buddhist, and has made meditation accessible to people of many faiths (as well as people with no faith). She is well-respected, wise, experienced, and has a great deal to teach all of us.

Cheri Huber, *Making a Change for Good.* This little book looks like a breeze when you first page through it. But instead, it is a very practical and deep guide to establishing a meditation practice. It does so by walking the reader through 30 days of meditation. Huber's focus is on the emotions that may surface along the way.

Thomas Merton, *New Seeds of Contemplation.* Merton was a Roman Catholic monk who saw his life purpose as nurturing the contemplative practices among lay people in the Roman Catholic church. Through his own practice, he also came to develop curiosity about and respect for contemplative practices in other faiths. If you wish to explore meditation from a Christian perspective, Merton is a solid teacher to start your journey.

Further reading

Brain and meditation: This is a vast topic, but a really nice overview that is science-based and accessible is offered by Brittany Fair, 2023, *The Neuroscience of Yoga and Meditation.*

Default mode network (DMN): The DMN is a large neural network in the brain that is active when your mind is not engaged in directed thinking. The DMN is active when you are day-dreaming or your mind is wandering. The DMN is also active when you are ruminating and feeling anxious.

For more information on the DMN and meditation, see Rachel Lit, 2023, 'What Happens When You Meditate,' *Standford Magazine* (https://stanfordmag.org/contents/what-happens-when-you-meditate).

Glymph system: The glymph system is essentially the lymph system for the brain. It was discovered in 2012 and the research on the way the glymph system clears the brain of waste and the impact of meditation practices is evolving.

For a more in-depth understanding of the glymph system, see Peter Wostyn and Piet Goddear's article from 2022, 'Can Meditation-Based Approaches Improve the Power of the Glymphatic System?' in *Open Exploration* (https://www.explorationpub.com/journals/ent/article/100422).

Another useful source is Simon Makin, 2019, 'Deep Sleep Gives Your Brain a Deep Clean,' *Scientific American,* https://www.scientificamerican.com/article/deep-sleep-gives-your-brain-a-deep-clean1/.

Lymph system: The lymph system is a circulatory system in the body. Lymph fluid moves through the system, picking up waste, bacteria, viruses and other extra material that should not or cannot be carried by the blood's circulatory system. The blood's circulatory system is powered by the heart. The lymph's circulatory system is powered by movement and by breath. It is a much slower system than the blood's system, though there is a lot we can do to help it function better.

For a nice overview, please see Ty Bollinger, *4 Ways to Keep Your Lymphatic System Healthy* (https://www.iahe.com/docs/articles/4-ways-to-keep-your-lymphatic-system-healthy.pdf).

Neurodegenerative disorders: Neurodegenerative disorders damage and destroy parts of your nervous system over time, especially your brain. There are many such conditions, with Alzheimer's Disease and Parkinson's Disease being among the most prevalent.

The science on the role of meditation and the prevention and management of these conditions is changing fast. A recent review of the science is offered here:

Andrew B. Newberg, et al., 2013. Meditation and neurodegenerative diseases, ***Annals of the New York Academy of Sciences.*** https://www.ncbi.nlm.nih.gov/pmc/articles/PMC5110576/

Pain cycle: Pain can become chronic when the mind has been trained to expect pain. Typically, this expectation reduces the amount of physical activity an individual is willing to perform. The result is that the pain becomes worse. The experience of pain is an important indicator, but it can be misleading.

For an excellent, brief and science-based review of the pain cycle, see Steve Haines (a neurologist), 2015, *Pain is Really Strange*. It is a short book that accurately describes the mental and physical processes of the pain cycle.

Patanjali (Pah-THAN-jah-lee): Patanjali is considered the 'father of yoga.' He is credited with writing The Yoga Sutras in about 400 CE. The Yoga Sutras is comprised of 196 sentences (sutras) broken into four sections; 55 sutras deal with meditation proper (the 'Vibhuti Pada,' vib-HU-tee PAH-dah, often translated as The Book of Powers).

There are many, many translations of this great work. A good one to begin with is by Shayam Ranganathan (Penguin Classics).

Sankulpa (san-KUHL-pah): A Sanskit word that means 'intention' or 'resolve.' 'San' refers to the highest truth and 'kulpa' refers to vow. Sowing a sankulpa is a way to build resilience and steadiness through meditation.

For more information, see Kelly McGonical, 'How to Create a Sankulpa,' *Yoga International* (https://yogainternational.com/article/view/how-to-create-a-sankalpa/).

Meditation apps

As for the books, there are many, many meditation apps available to you. These are some that I use now or have used in the past. Choose your own adventure!

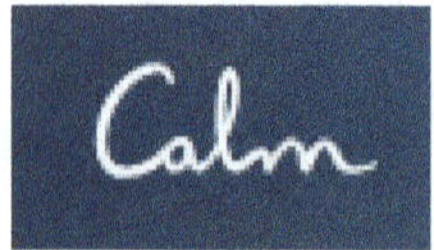

The Calm app has become ubiquitous. Some services are free, others are available for a subscription. The app offers guided meditations and sleep stories.

Available on iOS and Android.

healthyminds innovations

This app comes from the University of Wisconsin and is science-forward. It is free, though donations are appreciated. The app offers guided meditations and a ramp-up program in which the meditations are paced for new meditators and seasoned meditators. The program also helps increase awareness of how meditation is affecting your body and mind.

Available on iOS and Android.

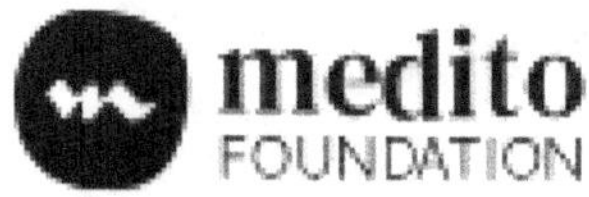

Medito is also science-forward and was developed by long-term meditators. It is free, though donations are appreciated. It offers guided meditations that are scaffolded for beginners and more advanced practitioners.

Available on iOS and Android.

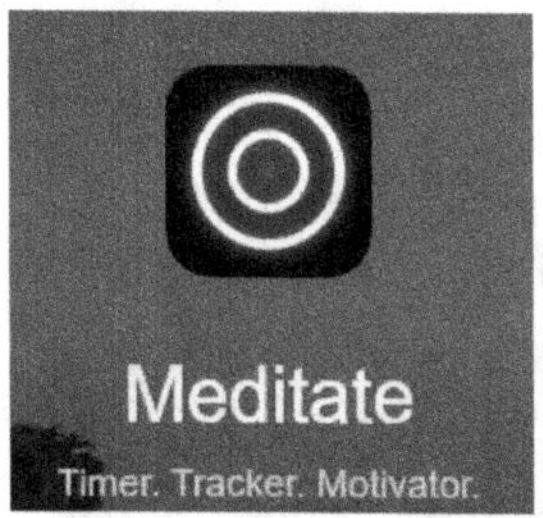

Very stripped down, but the Meditate — Mindfulness app by RhythmicWorks Software, LLC, is an elegant, free app (donations are appreciated). The app does not offer guided meditations, but if you do not want them and all you need is a timer and tracker, this interface is simplicity itself.

Available on iOS and Apple Watch.

Templates for logging meditation practices

Many meditation apps for your phone offer tracking for your meditation experiences. These are not great for me because I switch between apps depending on my needs, and sometimes I do not even use an app.

It is not critical to track your meditation practices. But it can be a helpful tool to either develop a habit or to remember and later reflect on things that came up in meditation. It can also help identify patterns of when meditation does or does not work for you.

If you find it to be helpful to you to track your meditation practices, here are some templates to get your started. Feel free to combine them, change them, add to them, or shift between them as time goes on. I recommend trying a certain template for a week and seeing if it supports your practice. If it does not, move onto another one (or don't track your meditations on paper).

Template 1 -- Simplicity

Date	Time	Length	Notes

Template 2 – Month-long check sheet

Month:							
Goal for the month:							
Week	Sun.	Mon.	Tues.	Wed.	Thurs.	Fri.	Sat.
1	◯	◯	◯	◯	◯	◯	◯
2	☐	☐	☐	☐	☐	☐	☐
3	◯	◯	◯	◯	◯	◯	◯
4	☐	☐	☐	☐	☐	☐	☐
5	◯	◯	◯	◯	◯	◯	◯

What went great?

What was a challenge?

What I learned . . .

Template 2 – Month-long check sheet, two sessions per day

Month:							
Goal for the month:							
Week	Sun.	Mon.	Tues.	Wed.	Thurs.	Fri.	Sat.
1	○ ☐	○ ☐	○ ☐	○ ☐	○ ☐	○ ☐	○ ☐
2	○ ☐	○ ☐	○ ☐	○ ☐	○ ☐	○ ☐	○ ☐
3	○ ☐	○ ☐	○ ☐	○ ☐	○ ☐	○ ☐	○ ☐
4	○ ☐	○ ☐	○ ☐	○ ☐	○ ☐	○ ☐	○ ☐
5	○ ☐	○ ☐	○ ☐	○ ☐	○ ☐	○ ☐	○ ☐

What went great?

What was a challenge?

What I learned . . .

Template 4 -- Reflections

Date	
Time	
Length	
Reflections	

Date	
Time	
Length	
Reflections	

Date	
Time	
Length	
Reflections	

Date	
Time	
Length	
Reflections	

Template 5 – Reflections on a reading

Book:
Author:

Date	
Time	
Length	

Section of book:

Reflections:

Date	
Time	
Length	

Section of book:

Reflections:

Summary of meditation practices

The soft landing

Bring to mind experiences you have had of awe when you were in nature or in the presence of something that spurred a feeling of awe. Choose one experience that has especially vivid or heart-felt memories.

Close your eyes and try to remember as much as you can about that experience. Bring to mind smells, sounds, and sights. Allow yourself to be emersed in the memory.

Hold that memory for as long as you like. Perhaps notice how this memory feels in your body and mind. Notice how you feel when you have held the memory for a few minutes.

Always feel free to return to this exercise when other meditation practices are not sitting well for you. It is a soft landing, always waiting for you.

Meditation practice #1: Tell your brain to stop

As explored in the first section of this book, this method does not work very well. You will NOT be able to stop your brain, but this exercise will teach you how active your brain is.

Meditation practice #2: Give your brain a stick to hold

Focus your attention on one of these things (your brain's stick):

- Your breath going in and out (breathe through your nose)

- A candle flame (in your mind or a real flame)
- Imagine waves coming and going on the shore

Just watch the breath or the flame or the waves as long as you can.

You will likely find that your mind wants to go back to working. That is ok. That is its job. Just bring your mind back to your breath or the candle or the waves. Be patient, be kind.

Meditation practice #3: Triangle and square breath

Please do not do this practice if you find that trying to control your breath is aggravating or upsetting.

Sit upright or lie down on your back. If you are sitting, sit in a chair or on some blankets on the floor. Your spine should be in a neutral position. You want the airway to be clear and at ease. Breath through your nose.

Notice your breath. As you do this, your breath will become more regular.

Scan your body and mind. How do you feel? Anxious? Relaxed? Uncomfortable? Exhausted? Happy? Simply take note of those feelings.

Take a number of these breaths and let yourself come into a calm state.

Now notice that at the top of your breath (when your lungs are full) there is a tiny pause before you let the breath out. And at the bottom of the breath (when your lungs feel empty), there is another tiny pause.

Thus, the breath has four parts, not just two - we breathe in, we pause, we breathe out, we pause.

Let those pauses happen. Don't try to control them, don't worry about them. Just notice them.

You can continue breathing with this awareness for as long as you like.

Another option is to explore elongating the pause after your out breath. Don't try to hold the breath. Don't allow yourself to feel air hunger. See if the pause can get longer. Maybe it can, maybe it can't. Just explore.

Scan your body and mind again. How do you feel now? Do you feel any different as a result of breathing this way? Simply notice.

Meditation practice #4: Notice emotions

Sit quietly and allow your mind to become quieter. Begin to watch your breath and allow your mind to quiet down. Breathe through your nose.

Now, bring up a good memory -- something that makes you feel safe and comfortable. Explore the sensations in your body and mind. How does this memory make you feel? What is happening to your breath? To your heart rate? To your heart?

Now, bring up a memory that is less pleasant -- something small, like forgetting something on the grocery list or a minor disagreement with a loved one. Notice shifts in the sensations in your body and mind. Take a few breaths here. Just notice. What is happening to your breath, to your heart rate? To your heart?

Come back to your safe and pleasant memory. Breathe. Let that linger a bit until you feel calmer and at peace again.

Meditation practice #5: Reducing the negative chatter

Note that this practice has a number of steps, and you might find it confusing. The bottom line is to anchor your practice around these five steps:

(1) Settling into the practice through the breath.
(2) Repeating your sankulpa three times.
(3) Scanning your body and letting go.
(4) Repeating your sankulpa three times (again).
(5) Coming out of the meditation gently.

Take your time with each of these stages. The practice should take about 10 minutes. What follows is one more detailed version that may be helpful.

The full practice:

Find a comfortable position to meditate. This might be one that feels best lying down. Whatever position you choose, find comfort. You will be in this position for 5-10 minutes.

(1) Come to your breath. Notice your breath moving in your body.

(2) Focus on your outbreaths. Make them longer. Count down from 10 to 1 with each outbreath. As you count down, you will feel your body soften further.

(3) Bring to mind your sankulpa. Repeat it three times in your mind.

Be positive. The work is already done. You are your true self. You are luminous, whole, uninjured.

(4)   Turn your attention to your body. Scan your body. Imagine points of light at each joint. Move your mind from one joint to the next. Let go.

(5)   Feel your body to be heavy. Let gravity pull on you. Notice the weight of your body on the floor or in your chair.

Notice the weight of your head, your shoulders, your pelvis, your legs, your heels.

Feel lightness. Feel that space between your body and the floor expand, maybe just a millimeter or two. Feel that expansion.

Feel yourself light, floating. Stay floating as long as you like.

(6)   Rest for a moment now. Just breathe.

(7)   Repeat your sankulpa three times. The work is already done. You are your true self. You are luminous, whole, uninjured.

(8)   Rest. We are now ready to be finished. Invite more breath into your body and gently begin to move again.

Meditation practice #6: Managing the information flow

Find a comfortable position to meditate. This might be one that feels best lying down. Whatever position you choose, find comfort. You will be in this position for 8-10 minutes.

(1)   Close your eyes and come to your breath. Notice your breath moving in your body.

(2) Focus on your outbreaths. Make them longer. Count down from 10 to 1 with each outbreath. As you count down, you will feel your body soften further.

(3) Bring your attention to your skin. Notice how some of your skin is warm, some is cold, some may feel pressed against the floor or a chair. Just notice and pause here for as long as you like. Let that noticing go. Come back to your breath.

(4) Bring your attention to your mouth. Notice the feel of your tongue, soften if you can your upper palate. Notice any tastes, any sharpness, and temperature differences. Just notice and pause here for as long as you like. Let that noticing go. Come back to your breath.

(5) Bring your attention to your nose. Feel the air coming and going. How does the air feel? Cool, warm, damp? Are there smells you can find? Don't try to figure the smells out. Just notice them and pause here for as long as you like. Let that noticing go. Come back to your breath.

(6) Bring your attention to your ears and to any sounds you may hear in the room or outside the room. Scan your space for sounds, not to figure them out, but to simply bring them to awareness. Just notice them and pause here for as long as you like. Let that noticing go. Come back to your breath.

(7) Bring your attention to the part of your mind that gives attention. For most people, that is a spot between and a little above their eyebrows and an inch or so deep. Notice the vibrations of that spot. Notice how it sits still or does not. Just notice and pause here for as long as you like.

(8) Rest.

(9)   Bring your attention back to the part of your mind that gives attention. Let it wake up.

(10) Bring your attention to your ears and sounds around you.

(11) Bring you attention to your nose and the movement of your breath in your nostrils.

(12) Bring your attention to your mouth and any tastes or sensations it offers you.

(13) Bring your attention to your skin and all of the sensations it provides for you.

(14) Bring your attention to your breath moving in your belly. Bring in more breath. Allow your body to gently waken.

Meditation practice #7: Move that lymph!

Move into a comfortable seated position or lie down on your back. Find your breath. Soften the space between your ribs and your hip joints. Scan that space for areas of tension and explore whether the movement from the breath can bring softness to those areas.

We are going to take three long, soft, slow breaths. On the first inhale, try to keep all the areas above your belly button still and allow your breath to move all the areas below your belly button, including your lower back and sides.

On the second breath, hold your chest still and allow the breath to move everything below the ribs, including your back and sides — all the way down to your hip joints — but have the feeling of starting at the pubic or hip joints and filling from the bottom up.

On the third breath, starting at the pubic bone, allow movement all the way up to your collar bones.

Repeat this sequence of three breaths five times, while using your calm, steady breath to quiet your mind.

Meditation practice #8: Walking meditation

Find a space indoors or outdoors. You need a space at least 15 feet to walk. You will walk quite slowly back and forth in this space, so consider a surface that will allow you to be balanced and comfortable.

If you feel out of balance, dragging your fingers along a wall or a kitchen counter, or using a cane or a walker can help steady you.

Here is how you do it:

(5)   Situate yourself at one end of your walking space, facing the other end.

(6)   Slowly begin to lift your right foot. As you do, say 'lifting, lifting, lifting.'

(7)   As you move your foot forward, say 'moving, moving, moving.'

(8)   As you move your foot to the ground, say 'dropping, dropping, dropping.'

Repeat with your left foot. And then continue across the space, repeating the 'lifting, lifting, lifting,' etc. with each foot movement.

When you reach the end of the space, you will need to turn around. Follow this process:

Bring your feet together, turn your right foot 90 degrees, bring your left foot to meet it. Turn your right foot another 90 degrees, bring your left foot to meet it.

You are now turned around and ready to walk the length of your space again.

Make every movement with kindness and deliberation.

Appendix: Yoga and meditation

Yoga is the cessation of the fluctuations of the mind.
(Patanjali, The Yoga Sutras)

We don't sit in meditation to become good meditators.
We sit in meditation so that we'll be more awake in our
lives. (Pema Chödrön)

In the yoga world, there is a lot said about meditation, but, to me, it often comes off as mushy and hard to follow. After reading and exploring various practices, I would like to share my current take and hopefully make things easier for those of you who practice yoga and find meditation confusing. For those who are new to yoga, this appendix may dispel some of the mystery around it.

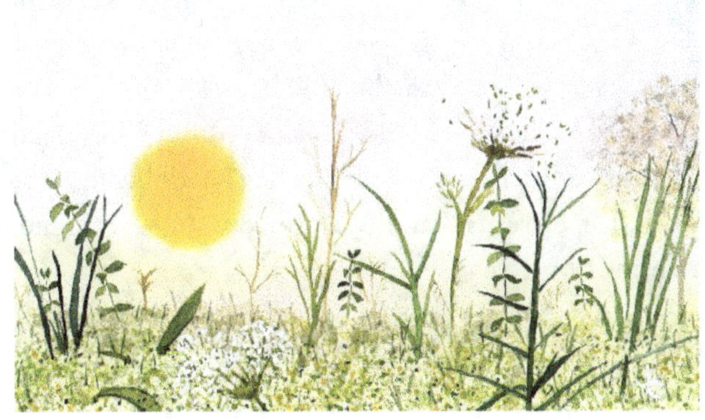

Weeding the garden

As I mentioned in the chapter on emotions, Patanjali (considered 'the father of yoga') speaks of memories and sense impressions as 'seeds' in our minds. While our seeds have the potential to grow into a beautiful garden, most of us have a lot of weeding to do. Those negative weeds are bad memories, hurts, things we did wrong, and traumas. They get in the way of true freedom. Like weeds in the garden, they crowd out, cast shadows on, or distort the positive and benign memories and impressions that are also in our minds.

The point of yoga is <u>to create space in the mind and heart so that seeds can grow, be seen, and be weeded if need be, and also to plant and to nurture positive seeds.</u> Our job is to clean up and make the garden beautiful. That is what it is all about.

When we begin our yoga journey, seeds often surface and start to show themselves. This tends to happen bountifully when we make effort around the ethical practices of yoga (see the box *Yoga's eight paths of effort*). We see all of our problems! We are unfair to others, we lie to ourselves, we are defensive, ... the list is endless.

We see many of these coming, and are not surprised. But some seeds surprise us. Either we have forgotten them, subverted them, or perhaps simply do not realize they bother us as much as they do. When I began a yoga practice, for example, a childhood injury came back to me during a yoga class 'out of the blue' in its full, emotionally painful force. I had long ago 'dealt' with it and believed it no longer bothered me, but there it was surfacing in tears during a backbend. Obviously, that weed had deeper roots than I was previously aware of and it needed attention.

Why yogis meditate

Meditation helps with both the seeds we see coming and those we don't, but it is particularly designed to allow forgotten and unconscious seeds to surface (both positive and negative). Like that childhood injury for me, these seeds don't easily come to light in conscious thoughts. The different mind-states of meditation can help 'subconscious' seeds speak up and be heard.

Let me offer a small example. My sister-in-law, Jill, recently encouraged me to start watercolor painting, and I was very excited at the thought of it. But the first words out of my mouth were, 'I cannot draw at all, so I can't watercolor.'

She laughed because she thought I was being crazily harsh with myself. But I was entirely in earnest.

A couple weeks later, I was meditating and a memory slowly poked up through the muck way, way, way in the back of my brain. I remembered when I was 12 and had taken a course in sketching during the summer. My aunt, who was a real-live, professional artist, was very excited. She wanted to encourage me and so she showed me a number of drawings she made when she was 12. They were excellent – really, beyond excellent! – and I said to myself at the time, 'I will never draw as well as Aunty Cathy.' And I stopped drawing completely!

Obviously, my aunt was acting from love but, because of the 'transitive property' of a 12-year-old-mind, the message I got was negative (12-year-olds hear things differently than young children and adults do – they have a lot going on). And, so, I have since always said I could not draw.

This all gave me a laugh when the memory came back. But Patanjali would say that since I was 12, my brain was saying the following words on autopilot: 'I cannot draw; it has been proven.' It turned a negative memory into a FACT, an important fact I needed to remember and hold onto to prevent myself from looking foolish. And all the time, the words were not accurate. I mean I never gave myself a chance! I may be able to draw. I may not. Who knows? And that was Jill's point as well.

Imagine, then, the force of deeply shaming or hurtful memories. They, too, put our responses to the world on auto-pilot; they ingrain FACTS that we must hold onto because we think those facts will help us survive. And maybe those facts did help us survive a difficult childhood or relationship or loss. But they are not actual facts, and they may end up misleading us in the long run.

When we are driven by these types of facts, or are on autopilot because of them, we may become overly protective, controlling, close-minded, sexist, racist, or a thousand other unpleasant things. But we are not living life in the now. We are not free. We are hampered in giving and receiving love. We are speaking our 12-year-old brains. We are acting out of fear and protectiveness.

Patanjali says, 'Please stop! Give yourself a chance!'

The Dalai Lama tells us that meditation opens our hearts to compassion and forgiveness. It mends us and makes it possible for us to be vulnerable and free. That is the yogic path. As we have seen in this book, meditation offers many benefits to our bodies and our health. But for yoga practitioners, 'tending the garden' of the mind and the heart is what the practice is all about, above all else.

Yoga's eight paths of effort

Patanjali describes eight practices or paths of effort (often translated as 'limbs') that share the common goal of growing and managing the practitioner's mind and heart. The term 'paths of effort' emphasizes that each of these practices is a life-long endeavor, and what matters is the effort we put into them. There is no quick and easy 'success,' no switch on the wall that turns on enlightenment, and there is no end-point. We just keep chipping away at our own growth.

It is important to note as well that although this appendix is treating these paths of effort as distinct and separate, they typically overlap. Movement often leads to a meditative state; meditation often leads to assessing one's behavior, and so on. The fact that a path is described as *starting* with actions, the body or the mind does not mean it stays there or that actions, body and mind do not affect one another.

This appendix focuses on the four paths of effort that begin with the mind. These are the other four, equally as important, with suggested further reading.

(1) Two paths of effort begin with how we act in the world - Yamas (YAH-mahs, often translated as 'restraints') and niyamas (nee-YAH-mahs, often translated as 'observances')

The yamas and niyamas focus on how to act well. The word 'virtue' is an old-fashioned one, but the yamas and niyamas center on two ways by which we may develop our virtue. The yamas take aim at our actions towards others and towards ourselves (such as non-harming and truthfulness). And the niyamas take aim at qualities we should nurture in ourselves (such as contentment and self-discipline).

For further learning: Deborah Adele's book, *The Yamas and Niyamas: Exploring Yoga's Ethical Practice*, is an excellent and accessible introduction to these two paths of effort.

Yoga's Eight 'Paths of effort'

Two paths begin with actions:	Two paths begin with the body:	Four paths begin with the mind:
Yamas	Asana	Pratyahara
Niyamas	Pranayama	Dharana
		Dhyana
		Samadhi

(2) Two paths of effort begin with the physical body - Asana (AH-sahn-ah, 'a position that is steady and comfortable,') and pranayama (prah-neye-YAHM-ah, 'energy/breath regulation')

These two paths are what most people today think of as yoga. Asana is the physical movement practice, which includes physical movements in preparation for meditation as well as the physical posture we take in meditation (usually seated or lying down). Pranayama is working with the breath or energy in the body. The word 'prana' means life force. So pranayama is NOT just managing the breath; it is broader and deeper than simply moving the air in and out of the body well. In her book, *Restoring Prana*, Robin Rothenberg uses the notion of the 'energy bank account,' which is very clarifying. Prana is our life force, our energy. Pranayama helps us manage that energy well -- learning when and how to protect and restore our energy during all the ups and downs of life.

For further learning: My all-time favorite introduction to movement and breath practice is Erich Schiffmann's *Yoga: The Spirit and Practice of Moving into Stillness.* Schiffmann also covers meditation practices.

The four paths of effort ('limbs') beginning with the mind

Pratyhara (prah-tyee-HAR-ah)	Dharana (dah-RAHN-ah)
Sense regulation	Single-pointed focus
Action: Regulate the uptake of information from internal and external senses	Action: Concentration on one object
Purpose: To allow the 'true self' to be 'heard' (and allow subconscious seeds to surface)	*Purpose: To build the muscle of focus*
Dhyana (dee-YAHN-ah)	Samadhi (sah-MAHD-hee)
Single-pointed focus on subtle objects	'Seedless' meditation
Action: Focus on (lean into) 'subtle' objects – resolve negative seeds and invite positive ones	Action: Maintain 'seedless' meditation (all negative seeds are resolved and positive seeds are added)
Purpose: Develop 'witness consciousness' and expand the role of the 'true self' in everyday life	*Purpose: Build capacity to integrate 'true self' with 'Atman'; develop steadiness and resilience*

The four paths of effort beginning with the mind

Each of the four paths of effort beginning with the mind has a different job to do. Each trains a different mental muscle. The goal is to tend the garden of the mind and the heart. The preceding table is a summary. Details follow.

Pratyahara

Pratyahara (prah-tyee-HAR-ah) is the management of the senses. It teaches us to 'titrate' or regulate incoming information and manage it once it has arrived. Sensory information can come from outside our bodies, but can also come from the inside.

Pain is a great example. A couple of years ago, while on a hike with family, I slipped on ice and broke my wrist. While we walked to the car, I was sharply aware of how much information the pain was giving me, and mindful of the fact that I could not answer the many kind and thoughtful questions from my husband and family about how I was feeling. I was consciously very busy titrating the information coming at me and was at my limit.

Meditation practices have been shown to be very helpful to manage pain. Pratyahara (management of the senses) is why.

Pratyahara practices allow us to observe how our minds and bodies change when we reduce or change the sensory input. Just listening to soft music after a long, noisy commute home from work can shift our consciousness. Our heart rate goes down, our minds become more relaxed, and our moods become more easeful. We are practicing pratyhara.

It is this quieter state that prepares us for the work of meditation proper, and we can invoke it by making choices about the sensory information coming to us. That is why for millennia there have been communities of monks and nuns that practice silence. Living with more quiet and fewer words opens the inner world.

➢ Meditation practice # 6 is a pratyhara practice.

Dharana

Dharana (dah-RAHN-ah) is the practice of building the ability to focus on one thing to the exclusion of others. It is often translated as 'concentration,' but concentration is too broad. I concentrate when I read a book. But in truth, my mind is very active while I am reading. It is interpreting, it is comparing, it is remembering, and it is being entertained or taught. My mind is NOT quiet. In this book, we have explored having a 'stick' to begin meditation with. The stick (your breath, a candle, ambient noises, walking) has the effect of settling down the rest of the activity in your mind. It is the first step towards one-pointed focus.

As you know now, one-pointed focus is not something we do easily. Our minds want to wander, they want to work for us. Dharana is a practice in which we build the capacity to hold our minds steady. We work at it. We fail. We bring our attention back. That is the practice: just coming back and trying again.

The purpose of the practice is, like pratyahara, to reduce the noise buzzing in our heads. When we do that, our true selves have space to surface, to be felt, to be seen and to be heard. Dharana practice is like turning on the light in the closet. There are parts of ourselves that are not accessible when we are busy. It is when we move into stillness that the closet light turns on and the true self can come forward. For sure, some of our 'seeds' may come to the fore while practicing single-pointed focus. They are our entry into the next path of effort.

➢ Meditation practices 2 and 8 are designed to build the capacity for dharana.

Dhyana

Dhyana (dee-YAHN-ah) builds on the muscles we develop with pratyahara and dharana. In dhyana practice, we maintain a single-pointed focus, but instead of the object of our focus being a physical thing, like a candle or our breath, we focus on what Patanjali calls 'subtle' objects. Here we allow our true selves to come forward and take center stage. We develop a 'witness consciousness.' This witness consciousness allows us to view our thoughts and feelings with a little distance so that we can notice that they are not our real selves. Our real self is the witness consciousness.

This can seem very vague and complicated. Let's not let it be. When my older son was two-and-a-half years old, he was in his car seat behind me while I drove us home for dinner. He said these words: 'Mommy, I'm thinking. And I can see my thinks.' The development of witness conscious, to me, is the self-awareness that was budding in my young child. We all have it already.

But the more important something is to us, the harder it is to exercise this witness consciousness. It is easy to 'see your thinks' when you are day dreaming, as my son was. It is very hard to see them when you are in an argument with a family member, under a deadline, frightened, or in pain.

The dhyana path of effort builds the muscle of the witness consciousness so that it is more available to us when the stakes are high. It helps us build the capacity to be in a sea of troubles and yet act with kindness and precision.

Also in dhyana practice, we begin to weed the garden in earnest. The subtle objects we focus on are many, such as the expanse of the universe, the truth of being, God, and the unending interconnectedness of all beings. And, while we do, we also have the opportunity to focus on humble, little, sometimes emotionally rife seeds as well.

In dhyana practice, we allow our minds to dwell on a 'seed' that is troublesome and simply observe how it affects us -- as if we are an objective observer. Once a 'seed' has been witnessed this way, it loses its power to put us on auto-pilot. It no longer has the power of fact. This shift may feel magical and liberating. When I witnessed the memory of my aunt encouraging me to draw, I was liberated to try my hand at drawing again.

Dhyana practice may also surface 'seeds' that were not conscious to us before, as was the case with the memory of my aunt. This can be scary (or in my case, pretty funny), but it is part of the process. There is no rush to resolve anything. Once a seed pops up, we can simply notice it and decide to reflect on it later when we are feeling more prepared. It is there. We see it now. We don't need to be reminded or harassed by it. We will get to it when we are ready.

> ➤ Meditation practices 3 and 4 support dhyana practice.

Samadhi

Samadhi (sah-MAHD-hee) is a practice and a path of effort. Patanjali says it is 'seedless meditation'. What he means is that it is the meditation we practice once all of our seeds have been dealt with, once our garden is flourishing. It is dhyana, but with no hard seed work.

Samadhi practices help our true self become the dominant force in our lives. During samadhi, the witness consciousness becomes fully integrated with the 'Atman' (the Atman, for Patanjali, is the Self that links all sentient beings, or God, or Timeless Witness, or whatever you call the 'thing' that you experience when you are in an extended state of awe). The muscle we are building in samadhi is this integration muscle.

What it feels like in ordinary life is that the true self becomes dominant in all of our actions. The Atman does not control us. It is not that kind of thing; there is no surrender or control here. In samadhi, we develop a kind of inner strength and steadfastness in coping with life. We become stable and steady and can walk through a whirl-wind with clarity and kindness.

This muscle of integration may seem impossible to even flex, much less strengthen. But my experience is that it is something that over time and practice, we can all flex and strengthen.

For example, witness consciousness, as mentioned earlier, is easy when we are daydreaming and very hard when we are angry or in pain. But what if through the practice of samadhi we are able to find witness consciousness easier to achieve in MORE circumstances, even if not all of them.

Our progress here shows when things that at one time upset us a great deal are now things that upset us just a little or not at all. Again, often just witnessing our own reactions to a seed is enough to take the power out of the seed. As we practice this witnessing, more and more of the things that upset us become benign.

Some even become gifts. For example, now I see that my aunt always wanted me to feel empowered to draw. And so now the memory of her sharing her work with me is a cherished one, rather than a confusing one.

Perfection is perhaps not a human trait, but growth is. And by focusing on growth, rather than perfection, we become <u>better</u> at allowing our witness consciousness to be the loudest voice in the room <u>as often as possible</u>. And that is yoga.

> ➤ The Soft Landing and meditation practice 5 are designed to support samadhi practice.

ABOUT THE AUTHOR

Jenifer Cartland, C-IAYT, RYT 500, is a long-time meditator and yoga practitioner. Retired from her faculty position at Northwestern University where she conducted research and taught for many years, she now teaches meditation, yoga, and offers yoga therapy in southwest Michigan. She is also a poet, with poems published in Wayfarer (Pushcart Prize nominee), St. Katharine's Review, and other literary journals.